# DISCLAIMER

The author is neither suggesting nor encouraging that anyone who reads this book should discontinue or change the way they use their medications. All information is the opinion of the author alone, based upon his experiences.

What the author has personally seen and experienced led him to investigate commonly accepted knowledge that, to him, just doesn't make sense; and he is now sharing his findings with you.

In this book, the author speaks about the relationship between patient and doctor through his personal view, not to be confused with how you interact with your doctor or health care provider. Please realize that the author firmly believes what you are reading in this book is 100% factual, but also urges you to know and understand that everyone is entitled to their own opinions, and is stating for you to do the research and discover your own truths to suit your beliefs!

*I do believe that this will be the most mind blowing book you have ever read!!*

## WHO AM I?

My name is Mark Gruell and I am writing this book because I have been in the nutrition/health industry for over 30 years. There are a lot of things happening to our food supply these days, and I would love to say the changes are positive, but "positive" is not a result that I am seeing.

Due to this extremely bad food supply and misinformation about it, we are seeing overweight and obesity situations that have NEVER been seen on this large of a scale anywhere, not to mention the so-called 'diseases' associated with high calorie malnutrition. I truly believe that if you read this book and follow it, you WILL achieve what you are hoping for in the arena of health, fitness, and weight loss. If this book helps even one person achieve a healthier life through its content, it will be worth the 30 plus years of research I've endured to write it!!

I call this The Body's Instruction Manual.

P.S. I firmly believe you will have a hard time putting this book down. I truly believe you will find the information massively riveting, to the point you will not be able to close it until it is finished!!

# IN GRATITUDE AND THANKS FOR SUPPORTING ME...

First, I would like to thank my father and mother, Phillip Gerome Gruell and Ethel Jennette Gruell, for giving me life and providing a great home to grow up in. I miss them greatly and I am so sorry that they will never get to read this book. It is because of their DNA, which was passed on to me, that this book is even a reality!

Second, to my loving wife, Tammi Sue Wilson-Gruell. She has been there for me over the last 17 years, and she has been the wind beneath my wings!! Thank you my loving wife! I love you!!

To my son, Joshua Phillip Gruell, this book has even greater meaning for you because you share the DNA that my parents passed down to me. I love you my boy and always will, you have made me a very proud father!!!

To my sister, Cindy Lee Kidder-Gruell, you are all I have left of my immediate family and you are so cherished by me. We just seemed to be the closest of the siblings from birth and I love you very much!!

To all of the thousands of clients that I have seen over the past 24+ years, it has been my honor to be your friend and to be of service to you!!

# STRAIGHT TALK

### *An apology for my straight talk—but the truth is the truth!!*

PLEASE NOTE: I would like to apologize up front. I beat on the medical doctors a bit in this book, but it's not that I don't appreciate them (because I do appreciate them very much, and we need them), so I don't want you to think that—in fact, some of my best friends are doctors. I just want the people that read this book to take the responsibility off of them. It is not the doctors' faults that you eat and drink so irresponsibly. That is on YOU!!! And if you read this book, you will know how to help the doctor become a better ally in your health care. With that being said, when you go to see your doctor, WHO pays? Because whoever pays is the BOSS! So if you aren't getting (or haven't gotten) what you pay for, you might need a new one.

For example, if I paid a plumber to fix my sink, it had better be fixed when I get the bill. It is no different when you see your medical doctor. If you say to him or her, "I wish to be truly healthy and on no medication if possible," then that is what they should steer you in the direction of. Now when I say steer, I mean you might have to be on medication up front, depending on your current health situation. But you can fix your diet—which is 90% of your health. Approximately 8% of your health is from being active, and only about 2% of your health is achievable through your doctors' abilities. In this book you will get what you need to fix your diet, and *then* you can try to become a bit more active. Your medical doctor should be on track with working alongside you on this. If he or she is not willing to do so, here is where you may need a new doctor.

I will not mention the name of this individual, but one of my clients had to fire 7 different medical doctors to find one that would work with him, and I also worked with him from the nutritional side. Over time, his doctor took him off 17 medications that he was on when we met, as he got better through his diet. HOW WEIRD!!

So in closing, I would just like to say that for everything you currently know about food and beverages, medical care, and medical procedures, I ask you to please be inquisitive. Be a truth seeker. It is amazing when people meet me for the first time. I have had several of my clients on their initial visit tell me, "Mark, if you weren't as thin and healthy looking as you are, I would have just walked right back out of your office." And you know I would not have blamed them, because if I am asking someone to believe in something I'm suggesting I had best be willing to do it myself. I would want any specialist I'm visiting to tell me what they're doing, not what they think I should do, and instruct me to do the same.

Then I can see the proven success of the suggestion. I will never tell you to do something that I am unwilling or unable to do myself. I will only share with you what I have already done successfully!!!

Now let's dive into this book.

IF YOU ONLY KNEW
The Body's Instruction Manual!

ENJOY!!!

## ALL RIGHTS RESERVED.

No part of this book may be reproduced in any form or by electronic, or mechanical, means including information storage and retrieval systems, without permission in writing from the publisher or author except by a reviewer who may quote brief passages in a review.

# Chapter 1: IF YOU ONLY KNEW: How to Lose Weight After Age 40!!

Okay, first - why 40 years of age? Because that is when I started to notice all the little tricks about weight control had stopped working on me. Now some people might notice this issue earlier in life—of just not seeing the weight come back off—even as young as 25 to 29 years of age. So, if you find yourself cutting back on calories or working out a few more hours a week, and you're not getting results or you actually start to gain weight and inches, this book contains priceless information. You are going to love the results I am sure that you will get.

I just spoke of working out in the first paragraph and I need the readers of this book to understand that working out is wonderful, but it only makes up 8-15% of your overall health. 85-92% of your health is what you are making your body's cells out of every day—YOUR DIET, THE FOOD YOU EAT EACH DAY!!!—It is impossible to fix your human body's health by exercise only!! Just a quick question here—why are over 58% of personal trainers/gym owners over their ideal weight??? I believe it is their misconception of how massively acute the importance of the right DIET really is!! I have been studying the nutrition/health industry for over 30 years and here is an interesting bit of information—In the history of this planet, there has never been as many gyms, fitness centers, workout DVDs, home gyms, and workout classes EVER BEFORE. So if the key to weight loss is working out, there should be absolutely NO FAT PEOPLE, RIGHT?—HMMMM. So why does North America have over 70% of its population in the OVERWEIGHT category????

Let me give you a what-if: Let's use your car as the example. Let's say you are a car, and you as a car need 5 quarts of oil to protect all the moving parts in your engine from wear so you as a car will run efficiently. We will call your oil your nutrition in this example. So let me pose this question: Would it be wise to only give your car a half a quart of oil and then take it to the race track, running it full-tilt for hours? Now I am assuming at this point everyone reading this book knows that would be CAR SUICIDE!!! The reduction of the oil from 5 quarts down to half a quart would leave the car's engine unprotected and it would destroy itself.

Well, this is absolutely the same in the human body. If you go to a gym or fitness center and your nutrition is not at 75-100%, you are actually destroying your body. When you do this, it changes how your hormones work and you burn muscle as an energy source and store fat more efficiently. The last thing you want to do is lose your muscle. So the answer to this overweight situation is simple—focus on your diet 85-92% of the time and your visit to the gym will be much more productive, especially as you age. Nutrition becomes more and more vital due to our hormones, and for me, 40 was the year I noticed my workout wasn't as productive. The reason that the weight issues didn't affect me until then probably had a lot to do with me being very responsible with my diet. That is why I am writing this short book.

So who am I, you ask? I am one of *those* people (a lot like Gary Taubes). We look at the existing research and we search for the REAL truth. Now, understand that if the real truth was easy to find, neither this book nor Gary Taubes' books would be necessary. So this is what started me on my journey to investigate cardiovascular disease. It has unlocked some amazing and startling information along the way—my father's death! He died when I was 13 years old, but fortunately for me, I was told by a health care professional that I would not live to see my 30th birthday, due to my own family's inherited health challenges. *I would die of health issues before my 30th birthday*–OUCH!!

I couldn't (wouldn't) believe them, so I went on a quest to search for the truth. And the truth I've uncovered has proven to do me proud, because I live by it every day. I am now in my mid-50s, no health challenges, at my perfect weight, and on— **NO medications**. So this information I am about to share with you has immense proof behind it, because all of the males in my family have had severe cardiovascular episodes in their 30s which ultimately led to their deaths. My father died at 37, middle brother at 41, and youngest brother at 34!

So how come I didn't die? It's this simple: I don't listen to doctors!

# Chapter 2: WHAT DO YOU MEAN YOU DON'T LISTEN TO DOCTORS?

Now, I don't mean any disrespect. The reason I do not listen to doctors is because I would rather take proper care of my health (the food that I put in my mouth) than make tragic mistakes with my diet, which will ultimately lead you to seeing a doctor. You see, only sick people need doctors. If you understand how to feed your human body, you would never need to see a doctor for health problems either.

Now I realize I just opened a major can of worms. This is because of all of the lies that have become 'mainstream' knowledge. Let me explain. When you go to the doctor, here is what happens: They order blood work, then reschedule you so that they can get paid for another visit ($$$$) to review your blood work, during which they hand you prescriptions for several new medications, three of which are preventative (WHAT A CROCK). Drugs DO NOT cure the problems; *they only help with symptoms.* So you still have the problem or the illness, you are just a bit more comfortable living with it.

Here is an example. Imagine you find some rusted metal on your car, and just cover it up with a shiny new coat of paint. In this example, the shiny new coat of paint is the prescription. See, no more symptoms. The rust is gone; everything is good now, right? WRONG!!

The new paint can't fix the problem. In fact, it causes complications. The rust can't breathe because of the paint sealing it in, which speeds up the oxidation process. The rust forms 7 times faster than if you hadn't covered it up. The moral of this example is that all drugs come with complications. They supposedly fix one thing—but what are they truly doing under the surface???

Here is another lie. Eight out of ten of those so-called 'required tests' are bogus. Those tests are just there to help pay for those elaborate hospitals! If this information is offending you, GOOD!!! It offended me as well. Now imagine having to spend large amounts of your own $$$$

and time (thousands of hours) because these lies are so well hidden that you have to peel back layers and layers of nonsense and crap just to find them. This is why you don't know that they exist. The medical establishment (hospitals, drug companies, and all affiliate companies that make their living off of them) spend $$$$—multiple billions per year—so that you 'know' what you know right now, which is JACK nothing about what they are up to. In this huge WEB OF LIES, you have to unravel a lot of strings to find out how they all connect. And I have.

This is a very big pill to swallow—I know. But, just look at the facts. In the US, we are ranked $37^{th}$ in healthcare by the World Health Organization. Not only do we rank so low, but we spend the most $$$$ by far for this lousy score. For the amount of $$$$ that is spent on healthcare in the US (multiple trillions), we should rank #1++++ by a very wide margin. Here is the best example I can give that we are spending our healthcare dollars in the wrong place. I live in a very small town. 70 years ago this small town had a five-bed hospital. Now, the 'Medical Community' says that they have made immense progress in the last 70 years. So, my interpretation would be that we must not need the 5-room hospital anymore, because everyone is so much healthier, we can close it. WHOOPS!!!!—So why did they make the hospital in our really small town 10 times bigger? How could these advances be real if we need so much more sick care?? Now, how can people live with these lies throughout their whole lives and never really give any thought to or wonder why we look and feel the way that we do?

Because they have us believing that this is normal and just the way it's supposed to be. Here is an example. About every three years, I have blood work done just to see how everything is going. Now the doctor I see knows that I will NEVER take any drugs, EVER, and we both agree with the arrangement; however, the last time I was there, a new nurse came in to do my paper work and the first thing she asked me for was my list of medications. I said, "I am on no medications whatsoever." She said, "Mr. Gruell, you are in your 50s, and the average patients at that age are generally on between 5 and 12 medications." She furthermore went on to tell me about 2 of these medications she recommended that

I should be on because they are preventative and people of my age should really be on them to reduce their risk factors.

Now I know she was sincere, but you can be sincere and be sincerely wrong!! You see, it's what she was taught. Just because she was taught this information, and the information was not completely true, doesn't make her the bad person. She is just doing what she really feels is the right thing to do for her patient!! Nowhere is it written you must be on medications by any age. HOW WEIRD that just because I am in my 50s, I have to be on drugs. WOW!!

# Chapter 3: THE LIES DON'T BECOME US

Now, understand these lies are not just in the area of health and nutrition. The public is being lied to about everything. Here are some examples:—http://rememberbuilding7.org/ –9/11 – LIE.

(This is one of my favorites) https://www.youtube.com/watch?v=P0VQqoJYhCE - College education – LIE.

Electric vs. gas - LIE. No new taxes – LIE.

Everywhere you look today (including social media and telemarketing), the lies just never stop flowing. Truth in advertising is now a fairytale full of twisted mistruths. I could write a 1000-page book just about this. But trust me; you don't want to get me started.

However, the vast majority of my life was spent looking into the healthcare system. WOW, what a contradiction of terms!!! Here is how I interpret those words: *If you go to a healthcare system, you most certainly **do not** care about your health, and that is GREAT!! And you are in luck, because they don't care about your health ether.*

Now I know, this sounds very bad, but please let me explain. Over 90% of human health comes from your diet, so this is what a trip to the doctor SHOULD look like. (By the way, a visit with your doctor should be a minimum 60-90 minute if done properly). Upon arrival to said healthcare facility, you would need to have at least a 10 to 18-day set of food journals to provide to the doctor. On these food journals, there should be the time you wake up and the time you go to bed. Certain stresses should be taken into consideration and, most of all, what you are eating.

It is truly amazing to me when a client thinks just because the grocery store sells it, it is food and you can eat it. WOW, how not true. Over 97% of so called food in your grocery store IS NOT suitable for human consumption. If you wish to remain healthy, that is. Let me help you understand this. Do you realize that in most gas station/party stores, there are over 100 different fluids you can purchase there? So why do you put gas in your car? Why not soda? It's less expensive than gas.

When I tell this to people at my nutrition lectures, they look at me like I am some kind of an idiot. They reply (most generally), "Well, that would destroy my car!" Well I've got news for you Jack!!! Sodas, fruit drinks, sports drinks and energy drinks are the leading cause of type 2 diabetes today!!!! Type 2 diabetes is not a disease; it is an eating disorder and cannot be fixed WITH A DRUG!!! There is a simple fix—stop consuming sugar!!!! It is amazing how many people that I have helped over the past 30 plus years who didn't understand diet, what is meant by the word 'diet' (the food you consume daily), and that any 'diet' works if it *nourishes the cells of the body.*

# Chapter 4: THE DOCTOR DILLEMA

Sorry I got on a bit of a rant there, but it is just very upsetting to do what I have done for 30+ years and seeing first-hand just how bad healthcare has gotten. But it would also be very unrewarding to be in the medical care field, *if you are a good doctor*. By the way, there *are* people that go into healthcare to help people and not just for the money. I know, I am one of them. I personally know several doctors that are just like me. But, there was a survey taken in 2014 with a question that read, "Are you taking this course for its financial benefit, or is it your passion?" It was found that 87.7% of students going to school in the healthcare field were doing so for the $$$$. Interesting!!

Now, understand I have no problem with a person making a good living. But I firmly believe that they should do great work for the $$$$ they're charging. I know this sounds like I am a medical basher, but I am not. When a doctor knows exactly what is wrong with their patient, they generally do great work!!

Here is an example. A patient comes in and the doctor can see this person's leg is broken. No problem, just do the necessary steps to set the leg then put it in a cast. WOW—problem fixed! This is what doctors are for. However, as humans today, we just throw caution to the wind *when it comes to our diets*, and then we think it's *the doctor's job* to fix us. Well here is the first problem with that thinking: over 95% of all medical doctors have absolutely NO NUTRITIONAL TRAINING, and the very few medical doctors that do have it have extremely limited knowledge.

Here is an example of just how limited it is. Let's say you and I go to the airport and I decide I want to become a pilot. So I take a limited course on how to fly a 747 passenger plane. It is a 4 hour class! So four hours later, I am now ready to fly. Are you going to get on that 747 passenger plane with ME?? Let's face it; it would be a safer bet for you to ask your plumber to make your next 8 layer wedding cake than to ask a medical doctor nutritional advice!! So having your doctor treat you for a nutritional issue is absolutely pointless. I just think that the vast majority of people have absolutely no idea of how to take care of the most precious piece of equipment that they own. Did you hear what I said? OWN! That is right, we own our bodies.

# Chapter 5: OWN IT: IT'S THE ONLY THING YOU EVER TRULY WILL

Do you realize that in life, our bodies are all we will ever truly own? Take your house for example. Some people really think that they own their house – NOT TRUE.

Stop paying your property taxes and see how long it is yours. I know people that put hundreds of thousands of dollars into their houses, but feed their bodies amazing amounts of junk. Some of this junk is quite expensive. But it tastes real GOOD!!! How unfortunate that they don't understand what is truly important in life. You only get one body. You must treat it very, very well. You can rebuild a house but if you destroy your human body, sometimes you cannot fix the destruction.

Now understand the first portion of this book is dedicated to helping you know and understand what you must be open to, and that is looking at things differently. Remember, over 30 years of my own research has gone into these findings. And here is one of my favorites. Can you guess which answer is correct? How many people die each day due to medical errors? A) 1,000; B) over 2,500; or C) over 4,000?

If you answered C, you are correct. By the way, please do not take my word for this. Do the RESEARCH!! The whole reason for me writing this is to massively wake you up and really get you involved in doing real research. Now you ask me, Mark, what do you mean by real research? Here is a great example. Answer this question: Eating Cheerios lowers WHAT?? If you answered cholesterol, YOU WERE DUPED LIKE EVERYONE ELSE. Here is the REAL problem—when everybody thinks the same thing, *no one is thinking*!

If you really look at the research, it is only the fiber in the oats that lowers the cholesterol, and the cereal actually lowers the wrong type! Let's just take a minute here, because I can feel your confusion. There are, as most people know, HDL & LDL cholesterol types. Now LDL has been stamped as the BAD CHOLESTORAL when in fact it has two natures. If uncorrupted, your LDL is more prominently going to be made up of type A molecules, and this is good. All A's means very little risk of heart diseases and/or arterial blockages. But if your LDL has been corrupted by SUGAR, your LDL will convert to the type B. Sugary and starch-filled foods are the primary cause and reason that LDL type-A will convert to LDL type-B. This also includes all foods that convert directly into sugar in your GI track. Here are some examples – breads and cereals. WEIRD!!!

Quick question, why would you want something as precious as cholesterol lowered anyway?? The higher your cholesterol is, the longer and healthier you will live. Remember when in the first part of this book that I told you that you had been lied to? Well here it is, THE BIGGEST LIE OF THE LAST 30 YEARS!!

# Chapter 6: CHOLESTEROL IS KING—SERIOUSLY!

Here are some FACTS about cholesterol:

1. Over 75% of all of the cholesterol in your body is produced by your liver. Virtually every cell in your body can make its own cholesterol if it has to. *So if cholesterol is so bad, why would your body produce so much of it?*
2. Cholesterol is the raw material that all of your hormones are made of.
3. You need cholesterol to produce bile in your gallbladder to digest and assimilate fat soluble vitamins.
4. Low cholesterol creates more health problems than high does!! The biggest and most well-known disease is Alzheimer's.

Now to get back on track.

We call this slanted advertising, and it is one of the BIGGEST problems that I have to face when getting my clients to have success. See, it all comes back to those LIES again.

When I first meet with a client who is trying to lose weight and become healthy, this is why it takes hours to help them see the errors of their current eating patterns and food choices, regardless of age. This is especially true when we start to approach our fourth decade of existence. That is the reason for this book. Now I know these last several pages have been, maybe, a bit overwhelming or even slightly confusing, so let me go into the nutrition side of things.

# Chapter 7: HERE'S THE DIRT—ON DIRT!

Here is the first hurdle when trying to eat better! United States Senate Document #264, 74th congress, 2nd session. On the second page, second paragraph, it reads (this is, by the way, word for word exactly how it is written):

> "Senate Document 264 was written in 1936 and submitted as part of a congressional investigation into U.S. farming practices." The leading authorities of the day had been sounding the alarm that depleted soil was causing a significant decline in the nation's health, evidenced by a steady increase in degenerative diseases. But when Congress saw the price tag on repairing the nation's farm and range soils, they swept their own investigation under the carpet.

This was a soil study done by our own government in 1936. – The study basically said that at this time, the soil was USELESS to bare quality plant life. So in layman's terms, THE SOIL IS CRAP! – Result? NO nutrition from anything planted in US soil. Now if this was the only problem, that wouldn't be so bad, but it gets worse. Very few people know that when you pick any form of vegetation from the host plant, whatever it is— tomato, cucumber, peppers, etc., etc.—it will lose 10% of its nutrition each day.

So think about that; most food in the produce section of your grocery store is between 3-7 days old when it gets to the store. But what if the produce person in the grocery store doesn't even put it out in the show case to sell it for 3-4 days, and then most people do not eat this produce the same day they bring it home. So you could see how this might be a problem. Because remember, there is no nutrition in the soil, according to Congressional Act 264, then on top of that, we lose even more of that precious nutrition in our plant life (vegetation) in the process of getting the food to the market. Let's say between 35% - 75%. Oh, and I forgot to tell you about the other problem. OOPS!!!

Do you know that they pick our vegetation before it has time to develop? Here is just one example. Let's use a tomato. Do you know that they ship them when they are about 1/3 of ripeness, so that they are rock hard? This is how they can package them, put into wooden crates (60-100 pounds in each crate), wire it closed, and throw it onto a truck stacked 6 to 7 crates high. Try that with ripe tomatoes and you would have tomato soup in no time. So, you ask, why are they red in the grocery store? It is simple; tomatoes naturally give off a gas called Ethylene when they achieve 90-95% of ripeness. – This happens in nature so as to signify that the fruit has completed development and is ready to be picked. So at the warehouse they just artificially gas them with Ethylene and POW!!—they have red tomatoes (not ripe tomatoes, just red ones).

Some people really have a hard time with the 'picking it before it is ripe' concept, so let me give you an example that might help you better understand just how very important this area really is. Let's say I am a doctor/farmer and let's say Mrs. Smith comes into my office and she is 3 months pregnant. So as a doctor/farmer, I know how important it is to get my tomatoes out of the field washed off, waxed up, put them in a box, and get them off to the market before they spoil. So this is the same technology that I need to use for Mrs. Smith's baby. I have to get that baby out at 1/3 of ripeness (that would be 3 months along). I have to pull the baby out, wash it up, wax it and toss it into a box and get that baby to the market before it spoils.

So I must pose a question. How do you think Mrs. Smith's baby will do? Well we already know the answer because at 1/3 of 'ripeness' or 3 months along in the 9 month term, Mrs. Smith's baby is not developed enough to survive. Hopefully this example, as ridiculous as it may be, helps you to really see the importance of your vegetation getting its full growth cycle and how truly important it is to your vegetation nutritional value.

By the way, organic is better, BUT it is very expensive and there are soil and time issues as well, so I would say to be fair you might get up to 5 to 18% more nutrition from organic across the board. Just a quick note here, 95% of all organic groceries in the stores today didn't even exist 105 years ago; they are all MAN-MADE mutations.

# Chapter 8: YOUR KEY TO SUCCESS

The reason that I am pointing all this out is because this information is key to making everything I will explain later come together and work for you to gain success. Just like when you paint a wall in your house, it is always best to thoroughly wash the wall first, fix all imperfections, prime the wall, and then paint. This is why it is so important that I take the time with you so you can get results that will last forever.

What I see most when I interview a new client is dynamic nutritional deficiencies. Here are some of the most prevalent signs that you might have a nutritional deficiency: Type 2 diabetes, weight gain, allergies, heartburn, acid reflux, low energy, joint pain, sleep apnea (all forms of bowel issues), most cardiovascular issues, cholesterol challenges, and thyroid events. This is just to name a very few.

Most of my clients are referrals. That comes from my due-diligence on getting people to know the *okays* and the *not okays* (the good and the bad food choices). There are food choices that make your cells thrive and there are choices that are so destructive that there is no hope for you, until you get rid of them. Now when I say no hope, here is what I mean.

I had a client who would come in every week. We looked over his food journals and everything looked good, but he was not getting success. After the 6th week of no success, I asked him if the next week his wife could come in with him so I could ask her what she was using in his food.

WOW, what an eye opener. When his wife came in, she asked if the beer and sodas might be the problem. Well according to his food journals, he was not having any. Come to find out he was having 3 diet sodas a day, and two to three beers at night to wind down.

Now, if this client would cut back on the sodas and beer and work on getting them out of his diet completely (and/or only drink them on holidays), than there would be hope. The first big problem is that diet soda is formulated to *make people fat*, and it also makes you insulin resistant. In layman's terms, it pushes you towards becoming a type-2 diabetic. Beer is an amazing story in and of itself, being that every ingredient in it (other than the water) is dynamically designed through fermentation to supercharge the carbohydrates, to create a higher inflammatory response. In other words, this produces more of the fat hormone known as insulin. *Remember, if you don't produce insulin, you cannot be fat.*

Insulin is the FAT hormone. That is why when a type 1 diabetic is diagnosed, they are usually very thin because their bodies cannot produce this hormone. But as soon as they start injecting insulin, they start to put on weight and usually get a bit chubby.

This particular client chose to stick with the sodas and beer, so at that time I let him know that there were no hard feelings, but he would no longer need my help because I cannot perform miracles.

The moral of this story is you cannot make constant bad choices with your nutrition and have a healthy life with a great figure!! There are disciplines that are necessary when you desire a certain result.

Here is a fun fact: Just two 20 oz. sodas a day is enough sugar calories to generate 30 extra pounds of fat a year—and diet soda is even worse, because it actually interferes with the sensitivity of the receptors on each cell of your body to use sugar effectively and efficiently. Now I didn't write this book to destroy your life, and I know up to this point it sort of looks that way, but please bear with me—here is where it gets better. Let's spend some time on what you *can* eat.

# Chapter 9: WHAT YOU CAN ACTUALLY EAT!!

FAT is the first category. I know, isn't that weird? Everybody says if you eat fat, you will get fat. Well with me and all of my clients, we have found the more fat you eat, the more *appetite control* you have. Here is why. Just think if you were really hungry! –For example, I have seen people who are really hungry eat two large burgers and two orders of fries and don't forget the large soda. If you were to weigh that food they just consumed, it would most likely weigh around 2-3 pounds, which would be the equivalent of 8 to 12 sticks of butter. However, I have never seen anyone ever eat even one stick of butter at a sitting (all by itself). Here is why: When you eat fat that does not have a carbohydrate or sugar attached to it, the fat will instantly produce a hormone called Cholecystokinin. It is ordered through the liver, which sends out a signal to the pancreas and gallbladder to send Cholecystokinin to your brain to let you know you are full. This automatically helps massively with appetite control.

However, if you make a batch of sugar cookies, there are two sticks of butter in it. So why don't you get full? It's because the sugar stops the production of *Cholecystokinin*—and that is why you can eat (the sugar cookies) till there are no more left in the cookie jar!! The moral of this story is mixing fat and carbohydrates, IS EVER SO BAD! So adding fat is a key, because appetite is what can ruin any program. You need willpower to feel good and stay strong, and then you will start dropping pounds like crazy. So let's discuss this in greater detail because I know you are having some trouble with this one.

First of all, let's define just what FATS we are speaking of: Saturated animal fat. WOW, hard to believe isn't it? Things like eggs, cheese, steaks, burgers, yes even bacon and sausage, butter, lard, and coconut oil. Now if you will notice, all natural protein foods come with fat. That is why the egg white comes with the yolk fat plus protein, rib-eye steak comes with a marbled fat cap—so you *can* mix fat and *protein*. However, at all cost try to never have protein or fat with carbohydrates or sugar. This is why fat gets such a bad rap. Because in the modern world, we have WAY, WAY over-used carbohydrates and it seems that all of the food that we eat today just seem to have these two foods (fat and carbohydrates/sugars) always together. That is one of the biggest challenges that I face, because when working with a new client, it is a constant re-education process to really get these two food groups separated as best as possible. What I mean by that is pizza is one of my favorite foods. I know it is not good for me because it has fat, protein, and carbohydrates/sugars, so I only eat it a few times a year. The same with sandwiches. This is a protein and carbohydrates/sugar—not as bad for you as fat and carbohydrates/sugar, but still not good to blend. Because when you mix carbohydrates with fat & protein, you get heart disease.

For Example: You get up in the morning and you have two eggs, two strips of bacon, one sausage patty, two slices of toast, and orange juice. So? That sounds like a good breakfast, right? It was, up to the point you added the toast and juice. Two slices of toast is 16-24 grams of sugar and just 6 oz. of orange juice has as much sugar as a soda – around 14-19 teaspoons. This is where we see the problems with heart diseases. I want to spend a little time here just because this is probably the first time you have ever heard this. When you consume sugar, the body has to get it out of the blood as fast as possible, because large amounts of sugar can destroy organs over time. The first place the sugar is sent to is the glucagon uptake in the muscles for quick energy; however, as we age, this area of our lean muscle becomes smaller through hormone reduction, and less sugar can be stored there due to muscle loss. This is a natural effect of aging. The other (or leftover) sugar is taken up by the body through insulin, and what cannot be stored in the normal fat cells (due to insulin resistance) is converted to palmitic acid.

This form of palmitic acid is the danger fat otherwise known as visceral fat. This is fat in the mid-section of your body around your organs. Later in this manual we will discuss the best, and sometimes the only, way to get rid of this type of fat. One good indication that you are creating a lot of visceral fat is a high level of triglycerides (which I find frequently). An optimal number for your triglycerides would be below 80 points.

Triglyceride levels are a good way of understanding just how much sugar and carbs you are eating; the higher the number, the more carbohydrates and sugar in your diet. Now triglyceride numbers cannot reflect damage already done. Here is what I mean. In the past, I have helped my clients greatly reduce their triglyceride numbers (through diet only). I had two individuals that had triglycerides over 1,300 points and in a matter of 6 weeks, they were under 100 points—however this will not stop you from having a heart attack or stroke once you get them down. You must KEEP them down. I have had several people come to see me, and they do great for a while, and then they just start slowly going back to their old bad eating habits, and – POW out of nowhere – heart attack or stroke. It is so imperative that after the age of 30, you really keep the triglycerides down.

**P.S. I would have them checked as soon as 18/19 years of age. It is very important for keeping your plumbing clean and working well.**

So let me start laying out a good diet for you. The first thing that I always do for my clients is establish what food they like, because if I try to get them to eat food that they absolutely despise, I will be defeated before I start.

# Chapter 10: NEXT CATEGORY, PROTEIN!!

Simply put, anything you can kill and eat – beef, pork, chicken. And by the way, you can fry anything in this category. Please use either butter or coconut oil. Let me clarify. Let's say I am cooking a chicken breast. I will first thin slice it about ¼ of an inch thick, and get the butter and garlic in the pan hot. Then lay in the thin slice of chicken breast. Let it sizzle for about 3-4 minutes. Flip it; give it about 3-4 minutes on that side, and its ready. It is the most tender and juicy chicken breast ever. If you like breading, just crush up pork rinds. Dip the chicken breast into the egg first (pork rinds will attach to the chicken breast more securely using the egg or egg whites). Then dip it into the crushed pork rinds, then fry— wow great stuff!!

Now back to the list: lamb, all varieties of fish (fresh fish, salt water fish, shell fish—for vegetarians and vegans I would have them use bean protein isolates, however I use them as well.

Let's continue: Veal, venison, duck, geese, rabbit, squirrel… hopefully you are seeing a pattern here. Oh, by the way, if the meat is fatty like organ meats, liver, heart, kidneys, brain—great! Eat that too.

Let's move on to vegetables.

# Chapter 11: VEGGIES—NOT WHAT YOU'D EXPECT!!

Most of what we call vegetables today are not really the best choices. The number one consumed vegetable in North America is the potato. This is just a big lump of sugar, because that is what it turns into as soon as you cook it. The only way the potato is healthy for you, is if you eat it raw. The minute you cook it, bake it, boil it... now it is sugar!!

So let me help you draw a mental picture of your steak dinner. You look down at your plate, and you see a T-bone steak and a baked potato. And you say to yourself, "WOW, what a healthy dinner." Now what if I took the potato off of your plate, and replaced it with a representation of the amount of sugar that the potato will convert into? So now you look down on your plate and see the T-bone steak, and right next to it sits two jumbo candy bars!! WOW, that doesn't look like a well-balanced dinner any more now, does it? Here is how I eat at a steak house. I have the steak, garden salad, and a cup of cottage cheese or chili. See how easy it is to get rid of the sugar, a.k.a. baked potato, roll, or rice?

Now let's spend a little time on this area: Here are the good ones: Lettuce, cabbage, artichoke, brussel sprouts, spinach, celery, asparagus, broccoli, cauliflower—a quick note here on cauliflower, you can cook it and mash it and it will mimic mashed potatoes quite well—kale, rhubarb, greens of all varieties, mushrooms, endives, leeks, and onions. Now remember, cooking any of these vegetables will reduce their nutritional content to virtually ZERO. Eating them raw is the only way they will benefit you.

# Chapter 12: FRUIT—THOSE LITTLE TROUBLEMAKERS...

This is a very troubling category. There are only a few so-called fruits that are low on the glycemic index: Cucumbers, tomatoes, and (in moderation) peaches and plums. All the rest have a high sugar rating. For my clients, I only recommend a category called berries. All of these are permissible. For example, strawberries, raspberries, gooseberries, huckleberries, blueberries, blackberries, boysenberries, green or black olives, and kiwis. Now I am not saying that you cannot have some other choices of fruit, however, fruit is nature's candy for a reason. It is virtually pure sugar. Now keep in mind that there is fiber as well, but in the vast majority of fruit there is not enough to counteract the sugar content. So for an individual trying to lose weight, fruit is probably not one of the finer choices.

Here is one exception: A real apple. So what do I mean by real? The true apple—unlike all the new "genetic freaks" out there in your produce department—is the size of a plum! Or for exact measurement purposes, it is less than 6 inches in circumference. If your apple is much larger than that, I would not eat it, because size does matter.

Genetic modification increases the carbohydrate, or sugar, and generally lowers the fiber content to our fruits and vegetables. Not only do they cost more, but they deliver far fewer nutrients. Just to give you an idea, have you ever seen the real banana? Not the genetic piece of fruit that we all like to call the banana: the Cavendish, which is a genetic and sterilized scientific freak show. The real banana has hundreds of pepper sized seeds, not at all appetizing. So, man came in with all their technology, and designed a banana in the late 40s that can bear no fruit, so every crop has to start through farming them by hand, again. They literally have to re-grow the trees from transplanting the stem of an existing tree. So unless you are an avid athlete and need a good carbohydrate to recover from workouts (for which fruit is the best carbohydrate), you should pass on the fruit. This is especially true for anyone with any weight to loose whatsoever, or if you are a type 2 diabetic.

Think about this: Throughout our history, fruit was only available for a short time, in the fall of the year. I have lived in Michigan all of my life, so for me it was primarily apples and pears. These are available in the fall so that we can eat them to put on a layer of fat to make it through the winter. See, there was a reason that we needed fruit—to help us get fat, but only in the fall of the year.

Not like today where it's available at any time of the year. So let me ask this question. Why would I pay outrageous amounts of money to eat something that basically converts directly to sugar (especially all tropical fruit - Danger!!!) which has no real benefit nutritionally? It just doesn't make good sense. So, from time to time, if you want to buy a piece of fruit, feel free. It's your money; waste it any way you would like.

P.S. I did buy two apples, and one pear this year, so I am guilty too.

# Chapter 13: NUTS & SEEDS

The best nuts for us health-wise are tree nuts, i.e., nuts that grow on trees: Almonds, walnuts, acorns, macadamia nuts, brazil nuts, and pecans. And then there are seeds: Sesame seeds, poppy seeds, flax seeds, dill, fennel, and cumin.

# Chapter 14: NON-MEAT ANIMAL PRODUCTS, AND A SURPRISE GUEST: CHOLESTEROL!!

Now, there is one other section that is still considered 'meat' because it comes from animals, hence animal products—milk is one of these.

**Milk** is for baby cows; it is especially formulated with high sugar lactate, and hormones to help the baby cow gain weight. That is why the baby cow stops drinking it after six weeks. So, why do people/humans drink it forever?? And we are not even baby cows!!

However, once the high amounts of sugar/lactate come off the milk in the process of making **cheeses**, now it is ok.

Animal products also include **eggs**, which are also very good for you, but don't overcook them; soft, scrambled or poached are the best ways to prepare them. Overcooking will destroy the cholesterol molecule, and you will not be able to receive the benefits of it. The cholesterol in the egg is priceless to the health of your body.

You see, the human body will make 2,000 mg of cholesterol a day. Even if you don't eat any, every cell in your body can make its own cholesterol, if it has to. It is the most important substance in the human body. The liver takes time to recycle your cholesterol, and every cell in the body has the ability to produce its own cholesterol in time of need. And all of this is happening without your doctor's permission—WEIRD!!

I could write another 1,000+ page book on the importance of cholesterol in the human body. But here is where the problem is: Remember what I said earlier that when everybody thinks the same thing, no one is thinking? This is exactly why no one thinks that there is a problem with lowering cholesterol in their body. *It is so broadly accepted as the right thing to do, we just do it.*

I overheard someone in the restaurant of a hotel once, bragging that his total cholesterol was 121 points. I was blown away that his doctor told him that was great!! Just a thought—if your body needs cholesterol to perform all the functions that cholesterol is responsible for, why all of a sudden now, just because a drug company made a drug for it that supposedly lowers the risk factor, do we have to take it?

According to the overall reports since the drug has been for sale, there has actually been an <u>increase</u> in heart attacks and strokes. So this would lead a person to believe that we might need to rethink this—and so I have! The real cause of all heart disease is... drum roll please... SUGAR!!!

# Chapter 15: SORRY ABOUT THAT SWEET TOOTH...

If you look at all the data as a country (North America), the food manufactures were encouraged and allowed by law (through massive payoffs to lobbyists in Washington DC) to add an additional 30- 50% more sugar to the food supply, and have over the past 35 years. When I talk about this at my lectures, I get a lot of questions as to 'what food,' and that is the biggest problem. People today didn't shop in the grocery stores of yesterday. If I could turn the clock back 50 years and take you all shopping, I could show you exactly what foods have had sugar added to them. But if you have no starting point, it's hard to see the result, which is exactly where food manufacturers want you to be—confused.

I have been shopping in grocery stores and looking at ingredients for over 45 years, and I have personally seen these changes. So I know that they are there. But I don't want you to just have to take my word for it. The addition of sugar to the American diet will show up, and here is what it will look like: the absolute fastest way to get a person fat is sugar and carbohydrates—*this is a fact*. Sugar and carbohydrates produce a forced response in your body by releasing insulin (AKA *the fat hormone*).

So, if I want to find the truth about sugar, all I have to do is see if I can find some fat people as proof that this is actually the reality. So off I went, to see if there was some proof and, wouldn't you know, I found it

# Chapter 16: PROOF IS IN THE PUDDING... LITERALLY

Here is the report from the CDC.

The first report I looked at was from 1980-1991. Obesity was around 13-18%. Now, 'overweight condition' is defined as people 30 pounds or more over their ideal weight. In 2009, average overweight conditions in North America were up over 25-41%. And you can easily see the trend line. 2016 – 73%.—Type-2 diabetes is up 48% and type-2 diabetes in children, which was not even- a disease 40 years ago, is now up 82%. This is what my research has uncovered, and you can feel free to do your own—however, most of you reading this probably won't. This research has taken me the better part of 30 years to unravel. I have clocked over 60,000 hours doing so.

Just as a disclaimer, the people in this CDC study that got fat— this was not their fault. The food manufacturers have been lying to us for the better part of four decades. These innocent victims were eating correctly "according to all the pertinent information," quote/unquote. IT WAS THE INFORMATION that was incorrect.

You see, it doesn't matter how good you do something if what you are doing is in accordance with incorrect information!!!! This is called security through obscurity. Simply put, you feel more secure in how you are eating because of all the incorrect information the food companies have flooded into the marketplace, on TV, radio, internet, etc., reinforcing your believe that you are on the right track. By the way, this is why your doctors struggle as well in trying to help their patients gain better health, because they don't have any knowledge of just how bad the food really is—and they have absolutely no time in their busy schedule to do this kind of research to figure out how to help their patients build a better diet!!

# Chapter 17: SO HOW DO I DO IT??

And now the moment you all have been waiting for— HOW to gain control of your weight and lose the danger fat: VISCERAL FAT. In the first part of this guide to a healthier you, I talk a lot about LIES. Well here are some very popular lies that we have to debunk. Who will this section of the book really target? That would be the people who are very serious about being the healthiest they can be, getting the extra pounds off that just keep piling on (for no apparent reason), and most of all, the ones who get it and are not plugged into the MATRIX OF LIES, who can see that there really are some very serious problems with the food supply— and the folks who have middle weight on their bodies.

Let me explain 'middle weight' better. Your arms and legs may have some weight on them, but you hold most of your weight in your mid-section. Now if this is you, pay very close attention to this section. It could be the biggest game changer for you EVER!!! When we are younger and our liver is brand new (not rendered toxic by sugar), this is not as big of an issue. However as we age, this can be a total game changer. How many hours out of the day should we eat?

You might ask what that has to do with anything. I am finding with my clients as well as myself that eating in a 4-7 hour window in a day has massively improved fat loss. It has also somehow helped my clients with irritable bowel syndrome—for some reason don't have it any more. Let's stop here for just a second: WHY would this eating pattern help someone with irritable bowel diseases? Well, think about it—the human body was designed to go several days without food. It is how our whole system is hard wired, just as the cave men seldom ate on a daily basis, due to being hunter gatherers. If they were able to find something to eat they ate, if not they went without, sometimes for several days. So here is what happens: Your liver, bless its heart, is the most amazing fallout shelter; it can run the entire body through storing and releasing, giving the body what it needs when it needs it, and to be absolutely healthy, your liver must be given a chance to do just that.

Let me throw in an example here: I want you to imagine that I teleport you back to the Stone Age. Where are you going to go when you get hungry? You look around—WOW no drive-through, WOW no grocery stores, WOW no fast or convenient foods at all—so it could, and probably would, be a day or two before you came across something to eat. And here is the best part: What if you had to pick your food from high up in a tree? Or kill it with your bare hands to eat it, which would be all the better?

So let's get back to the point I am trying to make in this scenario: You would have had no choice but to give yourself the time necessary for your liver to achieve a full release. This is absolutely vital to regulating and maximizing liver performance.

So, on a regular basis, we must allow the liver a minimum of 16 hours of total rest. It's just like how batteries can start to develop a memory. Let's take the battery in your laptop, for example. If you always keep your laptop plugged into the wall outlet, in a matter of just 6 months to a year or so, the battery in your laptop cannot function properly or hold a charge long.

I use the battery example so that you can understand how a constant feeding to the laptops battery, or constant feeding to your incredible human body, has some very similar effects. Say you get up in the morning around 6 a.m., and you get a quick bite to eat—nothing big though, just a half a bagel, which is only 60 calories, so you think you have made a good choice. But then on the way to work you pick up a cappuccino (or any specialty coffee with lots of sugar), and you miss lunch. At 2 p.m. you get a sandwich, and you're feeling pretty good so far, because you've only had roughly 800 calories. Than you get home at 5 p.m., you eat a little something while cooking dinner, and you and the family sit down to eat at 6 p.m., and later that night about 8 p.m. you get a quick snack, and at 10:30 p.m. you go to bed.

Here is our first big problem: No consumption of food 5 hours before bed time. This is what I have found to be true through all my research: At around 25-30 calories, the liver has to perform for 5 hours to do all of the functions that it needs to perform, before it can shut down and go into repair mode. The 5-hour window will maximize and help the body repair functions work more efficiently. But people say to me, "Well, it was just something small."

Here is how I can best describe it: Imagine you have a huge garage door, 130 feet tall by 125 feet wide. Now let's say it is an automatic garage door: So if I pull up to this massive door with a tricycle, will it not have to work as hard because the tricycle is very small? NO—remember, the door is automatic. It only knows how to work the way it was designed.

Just like your liver, when it starts it must finish, then reset, and this is where the tough part of understanding this is. In order to collect on the hours you sleep, the liver must have had time to reset, or your sleep time doesn't count. And believe me, the 5-8 hours that most people sleep at night—you want to be able to collect on them.

This is where the real work begins: Getting your schedule of eating to stop by 5-6 p.m.

# Chapter 18: THE WINDOW

Now let me reiterate, this book is for people that are having great difficulty in gaining health and/or losing weight, so I need to remind you at this point: If you are looking for a quick fix, this is just not the book for you. The rest of this book is devoted to people like me, who are willing to do whatever it takes, and are not into excuses!!!

Now that I have your attention again, let's put together a plan to get you into a schedule, so that we can successfully stop eating 5 hours before you lay your head down to go to sleep.

**Just a little FYI:** How do you make a Sumo Wrestler? Here is the recipe: Take a person, any person, get them up at 7 a.m., don't feed them all day, and then feed them between 8:30-10 p.m., and put them right to bed. Do this repetitively for 10-12 months and you now have a Sumo wrestler.

By the way, don't take my word for it, look it up—the fastest way to get fat is sleeping on your food. So the first thing we must do is find out what your day looks like. I will use mine for an example.

I get up about 8 a.m. and have a hot cup of tea—and remember there are no calories in the tea that I drink, so this doesn't start my window. Between 10:30– and 11 a.m., I will have a protein shake and several vitamins. This is where my window starts. At 1 or 2 p.m., I have my main meal—today it was a chicken breast, fried in butter, then I laid cheese over it and ate it. I also took my vitamins. At 4 p.m. I had a protein shake. That was my day.

Now understand that this is just what I do. You can eat anything you want for your main meal—you could have a pizza, lasagna, steak, eggs and bacon.

Also just as a side note, there is one other factor when selecting food that is very key, and that is protein consumption. Daily for women, 65-90 grams, men, 80-135 grams. If you do not eat this much protein, this will not work at all for your body. You see, your body is made primarily of protein/amino acids. To fix your liver, the proteins are absolutely necessary.

Now let's back to the 4-7 hours in **your** day, because the big key factor is the time window. Now I have done this with several of my clients, and it takes about 3 to 4 weeks to get a pattern down. Don't get upset with yourself for the first few weeks, just do your best, and if you screw up, just get right back at it.

Now using my example, put your own schedule in there. Let's say you are a person that is up at 6 a.m., to be to work by 7 a.m. So when in your day do you see a way that you can get to food? Maybe it's during a 10 a.m. break, where you can get a protein shake, or maybe some boiled eggs or some leftover chicken. However, if this is truly going to work, I would come up with a food plan, something that you have put together for a specific way and style of eating. That's why I have two shakes a day. These shakes are meal shakes containing everything the body needs, all the vitamins, minerals, micronutrients, phytonutrients, and botanicals along with protein complete nutrition. You will also notice that I use vitamins several times a day as well. This is because the food that is available to us, whether in our restaurant or grocery stores, doesn't have the proper levels of nutrition to meet our needs, as I commented earlier.

Let us spend a minute here, because this is going to be a big part of your success. The shakes that I use allow me to save time, because they're convenient. We all have trouble finding something quick that has adequate nutrition.

My specific shake has all the nutrition found in a 3,900 calorie meal, but it only has 220 actual calories. The vitamins and nutrients that I take are to make up for nutrients lacking in the shakes I take. This is why I use my specific protein nutritional shake, and these nutrients from the vitamins and other nutritional components—because they are not found in adequate amounts in the food sources that we have available to us today, in our barren food supply.

So now back to this window, here is how I work with you if you are struggling. It is best to eat in 7 or less hours in a day, but let's just work on finishing eating by at least 5 hours before you go to bed. This is the *absolute biggest gain area* in your goal to start losing weight and gaining health. Now keep in mind, if you eat a meal at any time in the day and take a nap, the same thing will happen. Let me explain—I am constantly noticing that a number of my clients say to me, well Mark, I stopped eating by 5 p.m., but I was watching TV about an hour later and took a cat nap. Remember, if you sleep, the body cannot use that time. So a 1-2 hour cat nap –will GREATLY stall your success. My advice would be to do something to prevent yourself from falling asleep. So now I am going to allow you to work out the bugs in the 'stop eating' arena.

What I mean by this is simple: Look over your day and see where the best time to eat will be, just like the example I gave you of myself. For me the best time is in the middle of the day, which is also my busiest time, but I manage to get it to work. And yes, it did take me the better part of 3 weeks to get it right. This is because you are forming a new habit.

See, what you are doing right now is a habit, which has left you with a result that you don't like or want—Weight gain, low energy, and health challenges. So now we must start on the path to the new habits that will take you to the place you want to be. However, you will see that these habits will be harder to come by, because the habits you have now are subliminal. This means you do them without thought. Because you have been doing them for so long, they have burned neural pathways into your brain. This is why it will take 3 to 4 weeks of seriously concentrating and meal planning to pull this off.

## Chapter 19: DECISION TIME

So, I believe that you have come to a decision by now, and have picked the best 4-7 hours in your day. The fewer hours in a day that you eat, the faster your results will be. However, to start seeing results, it will take 5-7 weeks before the liver starts really gaining traction. In the beginning I would recommend a 7-hour window. Then as you gain better control of your hunger, reducing the amount of hours will speed up the result.

If you have not picked your prime hours, please stop reading put the book down and put a plan together.

So let's apply this new way of eating. Some people find that cluster eating works better, where the majority of your calories are eaten at one sitting. This is what I do when one of my appointments with a client runs long. One afternoon my new client was a bit late, and she had a friend with her that had a lot of questions. The appointment was originally for 12 noon, but we didn't get started until 12:45. My normal appointment time runs around 45 minutes, but this particular appointment extended well beyond to 4:30 p.m.

After my appointment left I looked at the clock and said WOW—time to cluster. I had 30 minutes to get my food in for the day, so I had some chicken breasts from the day before in the office fridge and some cheese. So, I ate 2 small chicken breasts and about 4 ounces of cheese, and washed it down with one of my meal shakes. This is cluster eating: just threw down as much food as I could in the 30 minute and I was done for the day!

This is not something I do regularly, but to be prepared for anything, I have food available and ready, because if this is going to be the way you regain your health, **you must be a planner**.

On the weekends you can cook up some chicken breasts, steaks, burgers, even a roast, and put small portions of 4 to 6 oz. away, bagged up in your fridge and freezer. Then pick the best times in your day to eat them. —Here is an example:

Wake up at 7 a.m., and eat for the first time at 11 a.m.
Then you will eat again at 1 or 2 p.m.
The final meal will come between 4 and 5 p.m., to be entirely consumed no later than 5:30 p.m.

# Chapter 20: WHY WOULD I DO THIS TO MYSELF?

Now I realize that you are going to have to work really hard at this—I know, I did it myself—and to this day I still eat this way. I will never stop eating this way, because I feel **so much better**.

I was also afflicted with irritable bowel syndrome, and since introducing this to my nutrition plan, I have had absolutely no issues with my irritable bowel. Here is why: The liver is the organ that is the overseer of the entire digestive function, which is the release of enzymes to break down food. It is also the overseer of the pancreas, the gallbladder, and all of the intestines, large and small. So if you are constantly eating, it never gets a chance to shut down and recharge. It's just like your hot water heater—if you were to take a really hot shower for 8 hours, would the water be really hot constantly for that entire 8 hour period?

NO. And we know that, but our liver has limitations as well, just like the hot water heater has limitations, and must be given time to recharge between uses.

As I explained briefly in the first part of this book, when your liver has the proper amount of time to recharge, and heal, it is amazing the work it can do. Here is the best example that I can give you on how this works: Imagine you work in a factory on an assembly line, and the parts that are coming at you require 30 seconds to assemble and attach. So the conveyer belt sending the parts to you does so every 35 seconds, allowing you to keep up and do the job effectively and efficiently.

That is how your liver works too. There is a certain amount of time necessary for its functions to take place. So imagine one day at the factory, the foreman sets the machine to 15 seconds instead of 35. Just that small time difference would create a total mess, and by the end of the shift several hundred parts would have been missed. Any experienced conveyor belt factory worker can validate this.

In other words, activities that should have taken place didn't because the time necessary wasn't there. This is why it is so important for your liver to have the time it needs, the 16 hours of time off for repair and preparation every day. It is so precious to you achieving your health wellness and weight loss goals.

# Chapter 21: FLEXIBILITY IS KEY

Food and nutrition are very important as well, but you must understand for anything to have long term success, it must have flexibility. So please keep in mind that after you have mastered the food cycle that best suites you and your lifestyle, it is okay to occasionally break that cycle. I know, I and several of my clients have done it, and the great part is that you *really feel it*. I was very surprised, myself.

I really noticed was when, this one time, I ate after 8 p.m. I only did it once, *because my irritable bowel symptoms were back the next day*. They were not unbearable, but I could definitely tell. I was also bloated and didn't sleep well the night I ate late. It was truly shocking. So for me, I just love the way I feel doing this, and I am confident if you follow the eating agenda in a 4 to 7 hour window, and never eat less than 5 hours before you go to bed, you should too. I wanted to add a quick note here. In your 5 hours before bed, you *can* drink water, coffee, and tea with no sweetener. While we are on this subject, that is a great rule of thumb for all beverages.

# Chapter 22: THE BEVERAGE BOMB

This is truly one of the most difficult issues for my clients, because over 80% of the clients I have worked with did, in fact, **drink** the majority of their calories. And these sugar calories are very bad!! If you drink your calories, they are automatically in high calorie malnutrition status. This is very bad because this is where the fat hormone insulin goes into mass production, and trust me, with a name like fat hormone, you don't want that in mass production.

So no diet sodas, no regular sodas, sports drinks, even some bottled waters have sugar added to them—and by law it doesn't have to be on the label if it is less than one gram per serving. So let's say you buy a Brand X bottled water, and it has five servings. By law, it could have over a teaspoon of sugar in it.

So the moral of this story is, water, coffee, and tea is best for me, and if you stick to them without sugar added, you are going to be absolutely amazed!!

Also, if you need more help with food journaling, setting up your eating agenda, or food choices, my information will be on the final page of this book–. Contact my office and set up a consultation so that I may help you!!

# Chapter 23: YOU'LL KNOW YOU'RE IMPROVING

Now initially, when you finally get your window of eating down, and you have managed to discontinue eating 5 hours before bed time, you will start noticing a difference about 3-5 weeks in. There are two strange symptoms of your liver getting healthier. The first one I noticed at about day 65: Never in my life, even as a child, did I ever take a nap. But let me tell you, about the 65th day it kicked in, and I was totally wiped. I have never experienced that kind of sleepiness. Some may notice it sooner, and it lasted about 3 weeks.

The second symptom is some slow and slightly difficult bowel movements. This is not only normal but it will let you know that you have been consistent enough to get your liver functioning. This will not last more than 5 to 12 days, but just be aware that it is coming. If need be, I have suggested prune juice, or extra fiber, to some of my clients during this time, just to help you feel more comfortable. Again, this is only a temporary thing, and it will pass.

If you don't experience this, it may be a sign that you have not been consistent enough to jumpstart your liver. Just look over your food journals for any major errors or inconsistencies, and also your start and stop times. It may also have something to do with your supplementation, or lack thereof!

# Chapter 24: FINALLY—GRAINS!

Now as promised, GRAINS. This is a very tough arena, and here is why: There have never been more lies written about any one food group!! This has GOT to be the most socially excepted LIE ever, that grains and whole grains are good for you!!

Several decades ago, I tried fruitlessly to help people understand the fastest way to get fat was by eating sugar, which is exactly what grains turn into, even before you finish swallowing them. But there are some other properties that grains have that make their sugar content seem harmless!!

**Eating grain is very bad**. Just look at grain-fed cattle, as opposed to what cattle are supposed to eat (grass). The grain-fed cattle get fat fast, and the cattle that eat what their DNA was designed to eat, not only stay thin, but don't face the heath challenges that the grain feed cattle do.

So what do we do about this dilemma? This is a very hard food group to help folks overcome, I think because you must first be able to identify this gigantic food group. So I will better explain what grains are— Wheat, corn, rice, oats, barley, millet, and all of the food products that have these grains listed as one or more of the ingredients on their labels.

I really wish that I could tell you that in some oddly strange way that grains and all products made from them could in any way be at all healthy. But if I did I now would be LYING.

So I am truly sorry about the bad news about grains. Here are just a few examples of what is found in this group—bread of all types, cereal of all types, the majority of crackers, all buns, muffins, rolls, cakes, pastries, pretzels, bagels—the list goes on and on and on.

This group is the single most destructive to you. Not only do grains and all products that contain grain make you fat, but over 40% of the human population is very allergic to them, with autoimmune type diseases from this category. Here is an interesting FYI—in regions of the world where grains are not consumed by humans, there are no cases of multiple sclerosis. WEIRD!! But here is the biggest problem: How do you avoid them, when they are being engineered at an alarming rate into our food supply?

# Chapter 25: THE GRAIN CONUNDRUM

Consider that 97.7% of all food in your grocery store contains grain as one or more of its ingredients on the food label. This is extremely difficult but, wait, there's more—to add to this difficultly is that these grains convert directly into SUGAR. Here is an example: A slice of whole wheat bread has a glycemic rate of 70, and the number is to help us understand how quickly it converts to sugar in your GI track. Now, table sugar only has a 64 on the glycemic chart, so basically whole wheat bread converts to sugar faster than sugar does!! WOW–! Now add to that the addiction rate of sugar, which is 8 times more addictive than cocaine. WHAT?!?

What a category. I know, to try to tell you to live without eating grain sounds cool. But will it happen for you in reality? I am not sure. It is the single most addictive substance on the planet if you are a human. One thing I can tell you is this: The less sugar you put in your diet, the longer and healthier life you will lead.

# Chapter 26: DON'T TAKE MY WORD FOR IT

Please do not just take my word for this. Throughout my whole book I have been telling you to look for other good sources to get some information from. Listed are just a few of them, including, "Grain Brain," "Wheat Belly," and "Food Matters"!

These men have done the same thing as me, in the area of grain. I just did the research so that I wouldn't die of cardiovascular diseases like my family members have. They did their research because of their patients. Remember, earlier in this book I said there were some good doctors as well—here are a few of them, and there are plenty more, you just have to look and ask questions.

This is something that we sometimes fail to do when we go to see the doctor—please work harder on asking questions. The whole reason for this book is because of the tens of thousands who came to me *because* I could answer their questions, and help them to better understand how to be healthy amongst all the confusing and conflicting information out there. These are the same people that I am writing this book for. I have had thousands of people, for years and years, telling me I should do this. Well now I have, and I thank you so very, very much for your perseverance and your support!! You believed in me more than your doctors, your friends and in some cases even your families.

This book is very short, because I know when most people want to get started doing something, especially working towards improving their health & dieting, patience isn't easy. So I made sure you could read my book and get started on the same day.

I have referenced three other books in this, and I want to state that I did not obtain their permission to do so. I just feel that it is very important that you read their information also, so you can understand why I feel so strongly about getting the grain out of your diet. I must also let you know that these three authors have in no way seen, heard or endorsed this book.

## Chapter 27: REACHING OUT

If you wish to set up a 30-minute consultation with me ($100, and every hour after $175), referrals get a 50% discount if you or any one you know has a question. Please e-mail me questions with your phone number and the best time to reach you, and I will call you back with the answer. If you do not include your phone number to call you at, and best time to reach you, I will not respond to your question! ***Questions are free of charge about any information found in this book***. My e-mail: markpgruell@yahoo.com

Thank you again for reading my book. I hope you have found it to be very helpful on your way to becoming **the best you** that you can be!!

Made in the USA
Middletown, DE
14 September 2018